the little book of
DETOX

Published by OH!
20 Mortimer Street
London W1T 3JW

Disclaimer:
This book and the information contained herein are for general educational and entertainment use only. The contents are not claimed to be exhaustive, and the book is sold on the understanding that neither the publishers nor the author are thereby engaged in rendering any kind of professional services. Users are encouraged to confirm the information contained herein with other sources and review the information carefully with their appropriate, qualified service providers. Neither the publishers nor the author shall have any responsibility to any person or entity regarding any loss or damage whatsoever, direct or indirect, consequential, special or exemplary, caused or alleged to be caused, by the use or misuse of information contained in this book.

ISBN 978-1-91161-090-8

Editorial consultant: Sasha Fenton
Editorial: Victoria Godden
Project manager: Russell Porter
Design: Ben Ruocco
Production: Freencky Portas

A CIP catalogue record for this book is available from the British Library

Printed in China

10 9 8 7 6 5 4 3 2 1

the little book of
DETOX

sonia jones

CONTENTS

4

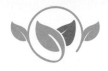

The word "DETOX" means different things to different people. To some, it might mean a weekend of no alcohol; to others, it's five days of smoothies or three days of green juices. Some even say that eliminating sugar from their diet is enough of a detox for them.

Detoxification happens via six major organs of elimination: the liver, kidneys, bowels, lungs, lymph and the skin, which is the body's largest organ. Foods and drinks that contain additives, colourings, preservatives, pesticides, artificial flavourings or sweeteners will overload or even damage these organs.

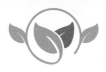

Going on a detox is a good way to give the organs all they need to do an excellent job of cleansing your body, allowing it to repair and to replace damaged cells with healthy ones. It's also a perfect way to kick-start a new, healthier lifestyle.

This little book will give you the components you need to put together your own detox program to suit you and your goals.

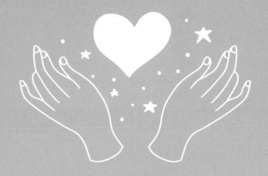

CHAPTER

1

SIX MAJOR DETOX ORGANS

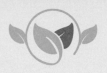

The liver, kidneys, lymph, bowels, lungs and the skin all work together to ensure the body can detoxify adequately. They work in harmony, so when one organ is overloaded, the other organs work harder to compensate, and this could compromise the whole system. Individual lifestyles can cause problems, overwork these organs and make them less efficient. For instance, drinking too much alcohol too regularly or taking regular medication put a strain on the liver.

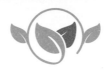

the LIVER

Your liver is one of your main allies in the detoxification process. One of the liver's many jobs is to break down substances into less harmful compounds, ready for removal from the body. By ingesting artificial sweeteners and food-grade chemicals, you are polluting your system and giving your liver more work – or in some cases overwhelming it.

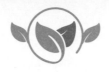

the BOWELS

One of the most essential components of cleansing is a well-functioning bowel. Including fibre in our diet helps to soften stools, preventing constipation, which speeds up the transition of waste. This drastically cuts down autointoxication, where the longer waste stays in the bowel, the more waste is reabsorbed. Fibre also feeds the correct bowel flora, helping to reduce your toxic load.

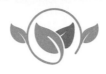

the KIDNEYS

One of the keys to cleansing is getting hydrated. However, caffeinated drinks such as coffee, tea, alcohol and soft drinks function as diuretics, putting unnecessary strain on the delicate cells of the kidneys. These dehydrating drinks won't help in the detox process.

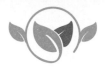

the LYMPH

The lymph helps to remove waste from the body, and it is part of the immune system. Unlike the circulatory system, it has no pump, so it can quickly become sluggish and congested.

As most people lead sedentary lives, part of the detox process will mean moving more, because the muscles encourage a better flow of lymph.

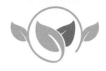

the SKIN

The skin is the largest detox organ, and we need to encourage the skin to function better by ensuring that we use the best products on it. (We will talk more about skin products later.) Sweating is essential, as is exfoliation and getting some sun – although not too much.

They say skin often mirrors the state of your inner health, so the good news is the skin will look and function better after a detox.

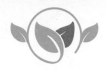

the LUNGS

Our lungs remove waste from the body through breathing. Shallow breathing, bad posture and stress significantly affect the function of the lungs. Most of us spend most of our time inside, so it is essential to get out in the fresh air regularly and to take brisk walks.

Taking in more air will help every cell detox more efficiently.

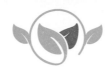

"Health is the greatest
gift, contentment
the greatest wealth,
faithfulness the best
relationship."

GAUTAMA BUDDHA

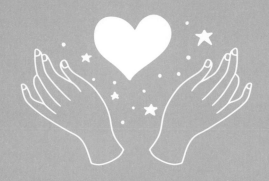

CHAPTER
2

HYDRATION

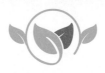

Did you know?

Most people confuse the sensation of thirst with hunger, often going for a snack when, in fact, they should be drinking something hydrating. Many people just don't drink enough water or hydrating drinks, even though everyone would agree that water is good for them. It may sound too simple, but if you want to detox, you will need to start hydrating to enable cells to flush out toxins. My patients often give one of the following four excuses for not drinking enough water:

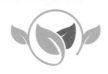

"I forget."

"I don't like the taste."

"Water makes me feel sick."

*"I worry that I might
   drink too much at a time."*

Let's address these now...

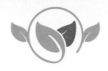

"I forget."

If you have trouble remembering to keep hydrated, make sure to take a bottle of water to work with you and keep it on your desk within eyesight.

If you work from home, keep a bottle in the kitchen to remind you. Leave notes to yourself, ask a friend, set an alarm clock or even stick a note on your head. Whatever works for you!

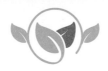

"*I don't like the taste.*"

If it's the flavour that's bothering you, try adding a squeeze of fresh lemon to your water, as that makes all the difference to the taste.

If your tap water tastes terrible, consider filtering it first, with a jug that sits in the fridge or by fitting a filter to your water supply – you'll notice a considerable change in taste and smell.

Bottled water varies significantly, but the higher-quality water tastes the best.

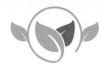

"Water makes me feel sick."

If water makes you feel nauseous, try
sipping a little throughout the day, or
you may find hot water with a bit of fresh
ginger is the answer. This works really
well for those who feel sick, as ginger
has been used for centuries to combat
nausea. Hot water and peppermint can
be good too.

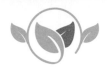

"I worry that I might drink too much at a time."

Drinking lots of water often coincides with a person going on a sudden health kick. A typical scenario is deciding to give up tea, coffee or fizzy drinks overnight in favour of water. This is not a brilliant idea. The withdrawal symptoms will make you feel terrible, so it is better to do it gradually.

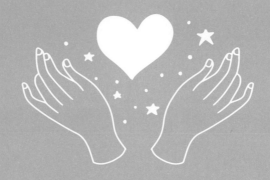

CHAPTER
3

FRUIT and VEGETABLES

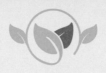

Fruits and vegetables are a fundamental part of any detox plan and of any healthy diet. All fresh fruit and vegetables contain enzymes, plant compounds, vitamins and minerals. I have highlighted a few of them below since there are too many to mention them all. All fresh produce is good for you, and you should aim to eat and drink about nine or more portions a day while you are detoxing. The five-a-day that is generally recommended is a daily minimum. Overcooking will destroy enzymes and some nutrients, so if you must boil vegetables, make sure you also drink the water.

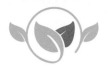

APPLE

Apples are high in antioxidants, flavonoids and fibre, especially a specific fibre called pectin.

All fibre is good at cleansing, but pectin is particularly useful for cleansing the colon and flushing toxins out of your system. Apples are also particularly good at helping to cleanse your liver and gallbladder.

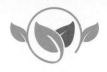

ARTICHOKE

Artichokes increase bile production. One of the jobs of bile is to transport toxins and debris, such as dead red blood cells, into the bowel, ready to be removed from the body.

Betanin, which is found in artichokes, helps the liver break down fatty acids more efficiently, protecting the liver and allowing it to function better.

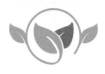

ASPARAGUS

We all know when we eat asparagus; it's not long before our pee smells strange. Research has discovered that compounds found in asparagus stimulate the kidneys and bowels to excrete more toxins. Asparagus is packed with a plant compound called rutin.

Rutin is also found in buckwheat, and it encourages the health of the tiny capillaries.

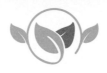

AVOCADO

Our hangovers get worse as we get older, due to decreasing levels of glutathione, but avocado combines with fat-soluble toxins to turn them into water-soluble ones, which are easier for the body to remove as they are less harmful.

Research has shown that people with higher levels of glutathione were generally healthier and less likely to suffer from "the morning after".

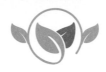

BEETROOT

Beetroot has been used for centuries as a purifying blood-cleanser, so it is also beneficial for the liver. Beetroot contains the fibre pectin, which is particularly good for cleansing the colon and flushing toxins out of the body.

Beetroot also contains methionine, helping to neutralize toxins. This also helps speed up circulation and metabolism.

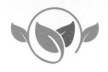

CARROT

Carrots are a rich source of alpha-carotene and beta-carotene, and the liver converts them to vitamin A when needed.

Carrots also seem to have the ability to bind with heavy metal ready for excretion. Plant compounds in carrots can help reduce cholesterol, and this, in turn, promotes better circulation.

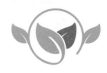

CUCUMBER

Cucumbers help cleanse the entire system, aiding in digestion, helping reduce fluid retention, and they have a very mild laxative action. Cucumbers help flush the kidneys and the bladder. They also help dissolve uric acid build-up.

They are excellent for hydrating, which is a necessary component of detoxing.

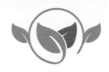

CABBAGE

Cabbage is well known for healing the digestive lining in general. It is rich in vitamin U, named U as it was found to be good for healing ulcers. It is a also a highly effective bowel cleanser.

Varieties include white, red and green cabbage plus spring cabbage and Chinese cabbage.

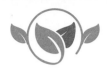

COURGETTE/ ZUCCHINI

Courgettes encourage healthy digestion, generally detoxify and lower cholesterol. They have mild laxative and diuretic properties, and they help the liver to function better, aiding metabolism, hydration and stabilizing blood sugar levels. They can be dark green or yellow, and they belong to the same family as the marrow, squash and pumpkin.

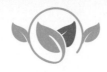

LEMON

No detox program would be complete without fresh lemons, with their familiar zesty, clean taste. Lemon is renowned for being very alkaline-forming in the body and extremely good for the liver, which is one of the major detoxifying organs.

Due to poor diet choices, most people's systems are too acidic, so lemons are especially useful.

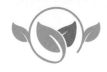

PARSLEY

Parsley is a reliable source of minerals and chlorophyll, making it a potent cleanser. It is also a good blood purifier that is great for stimulating the bowels, and it aids the kidneys, helping to solve fluid-retention problems. It reduces coagulants, too, and helps to clear and prevent kidney stones.

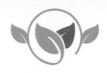

PASSIONFRUIT

Passionfruit has an amazing aroma, and a fresh, clean and somewhat lemony taste. As well as soothing the digestive tract, it is rich in vitamin C, antioxidants and magnesium.

Many people just don't get enough magnesium, which is needed for many functions, but especially for the bowel, the nervous system and muscles.

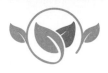

PRUNE

Prunes are a rich source of antioxidants. They also contain tartaric acid, which is a mild natural laxative, and dihydroxyphenyl isatin, which encourages peristalsis – the regular contractions of the bowels.

Together these two compounds promote bowel movements, reducing the time that any waste matter stays in the colon. This limits the time toxins sit around, being reabsorbed into the system.

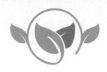

SEAWEED

Properties in sea vegetables help bind with radioactive waste, making them less harmful. This type of waste can come from the soil that food is grown in. Seaweed is a rich source of iron, calcium, iodine and magnesium, all of which are needed in the detox process.

Alginates found in these vegetables bind with heavy metals, easing their excretion from the body.

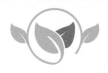

DARK GREEN LEAVES

Dark green leaves such as kale, collard, cabbage, watercress, dark green lettuce, spinach and the like are all reliable sources of minerals and chlorophyll. Chlorophyll is a powerful cleanser, a particularly good blood purifier, and it is excellent for stimulating the bowels. It also helps to strengthen the blood, especially if you are prone to anaemia.

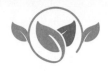

WATERCRESS

Watercress is rich in chlorophyll, which helps fortify red blood cells and encourages better circulation, which in turn enables every cell to function at its best. It is thought watercress contains enzymes that promote detoxification.

Research has shown that when smokers were given six to eight ounces of watercress every day, they excreted higher levels than usual of carcinogens in their urine.

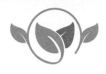

"He who has health
has hope and he
who has hope has
everything."

ARABIAN PROVERB

detox
DRINKS

Besides making juices and smoothies
made from fresh fruit, vegetables
and herbs, there are plenty of other
drinks that can help the detox process.
All of these are made from easy-to-
find ingredients, such as apple cider
vinegar, herbs or spices. Some drinks
are taken hot, others cold. These
drinks will help the detoxing process
without you needing to drink too
many fruit-based juices or smoothies.

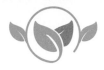

APPLE CIDER VINEGAR DRINK

- 1oz/30ml raw, unfiltered organic apple cider vinegar
- 8oz/230ml purified or bottled water
- 1 tsp honey or maple syrup
- Dash of lemon juice (optional)

Natural apple cider contains enzymes and high doses of potassium. It helps to balance the correct level of acid and alkali, and it helps feed the good bacteria in your gut.

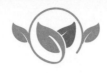

COCONUT WATER

Coconut water has a natural balance of sodium, potassium, calcium and magnesium, making it a wonderfully healthy electrolyte drink. In other words, it is very hydrating. Coconut water can help every cell in the body to function better by being able to hydrate and flush out any debris. It also helps the circulation and increases oxygen to the cells.

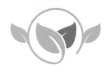

KOMBUCHA

This is a fermented drink made by adding specific strains of bacteria, yeast and sugar to green tea and allowing it to ferment for a week or more. Kombucha can help to eliminate unwanted toxins from your gut, and the probiotic nature of this drink improves the health of your intestinal cells, boosts your immune system and increases detoxification. Kombucha can be bought in many flavours or made at home with a starter.

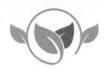

KEFIR WATER

Kefir is a fermented drink with live microorganisms that help replace good bacteria that are lost after taking a dose of antibiotics.

For the bowels to function correctly, they need the correct bowel flora, and "good bacteria" has a profound effect on our overall health and helps us avoid constipation. Kefir water can be bought in various flavours or made at home.

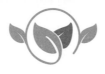

COCONUT KEFIR

This is a beverage made from kefir grains and coconut water. The "good bacteria" it contains will cleanse the intestines, detoxify the gut, reduce flatulence, control bowel movement and provide nourishment.

Kefir also boosts the immune system and improves the metabolic system, leading to a healthier life with more energy.

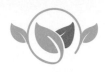

LEMON, CAYENNE PEPPER and HONEY DRINK

- 10oz/300ml water
- 2 tbsp fresh organic lemon juice
- 1 tbsp honey
- Pinch or more of cayenne pepper

This drink is the main component of the *Master Cleanse Diet* (also called the *Lemonade Diet* or the *Beyoncé Diet*). Drink it in the morning, and the combination of these ingredients will have a powerful cleansing effect on the body.

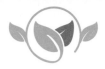

LEMON
and GINGER DRINK

- 1 unwaxed or organic lemon
- Small piece of fresh ginger
- ½ tsp powdered turmeric
- Pinch of cayenne pepper
- 35oz/1 litre water

Chop up the ginger and lemon, place it in the water, bring to the boil and switch off the heat immediately. Add turmeric and cayenne to taste. Strain and drink at room temperature, keeping any leftovers in the fridge.

WATERMELON DRINK

Watermelon is exceptionally alkaline-forming in the body, as is a lot of fruit. This is important because an acidic body can't detox efficiently. Make sure to incorporate the pale flesh of the watermelon that is close to the rind, which is rich in nutrients that help the liver and the kidneys do a better job. Watermelon is good for hydrating, and it has high levels of other nutrients. To make the drink, simply zap some watermelon in a blender and add a little ginger or lemon.

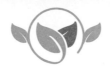

HOMEMADE VEGETABLE STOCK

This is an easy recipe that costs next to nothing to make. When you have some clean peelings from any of your vegetables, collect them for two or three days, keeping them in the fridge until ready to use. Place them all in a saucepan and cover with water. Add some onions, chilli, garlic, herbs, ginger and pepper. Bring to the boil, then simmer for 30 minutes. Sieve out all the vegetables and store the stock in the refrigerator for up to three days or in the freezer for up to three months.

detox
TEA

Herbal preparations have been made for centuries to help treat all sorts of ailments and to help the body eliminate toxins. The simplest way to take herbs is in a tea, which is called an infusion, usually made with the leaf of the plant or the flower head. Decoctions (simmering the plant parts in a pan with water) are used for the tough parts of the plant, like the seeds or bark. The general rule of thumb is one teaspoon per cup of water. You can always make a batch and keep it in the fridge until needed.

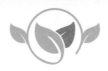

DANDELION LEAF and ROOT TEA

Dandelions are a reliable source of vitamin A, potassium, iron and calcium. Dandelion leaf helps the kidneys detox while the root supports the liver.

Add four teaspoons of dandelion root to five cups of water and bring to the boil, then simmer for five minutes. Turn off the heat and add four teaspoons of dandelion leaves, then leave to steep for ten minutes. Drink one cup a day, keeping any leftovers in the fridge.

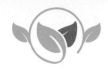

FENNEL SEED TEA

The chemical compound anethole in fennel helps detox both the stomach and the liver.

Use one teaspoon of seeds per cup of boiled water, steep for ten minutes and drink three times a day to encourage elimination through the urinary and intestinal tracts.

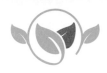

MILK THISTLE TEA

It has been well known for centuries that milk thistle helps the liver regenerate and detox. It also has potent antioxidants, which is what you need when you want to do a liver cleanse.

Milk thistle also boosts bile evacuation and repairs liver damage. Put one teaspoon of dried milk thistle into a cup of boiled water and infuse for five to ten minutes. Drink once a day.

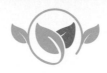

SAGE TEA

Sleep is essential for the body to function, and sage will help you sleep better. Sage also enhances the memory and restores energy, and has a tonic effect on the liver that helps the body to detox more efficiently.

To make sage tea, steep one to two teaspoons of sage in a cup of boiled water for five to eight minutes. Drink one cup three times a day for a few days (avoid taking it long term).

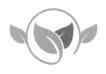

"Lack of activity destroys the good condition of every human being, while movement and methodical physical exercise save it and preserve it."

PLATO

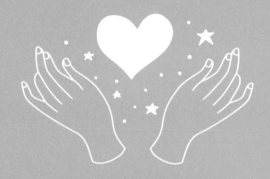

CHAPTER

4

LIVE
ENZYMES and
BACTERIA

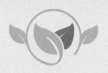

Both live enzymes and certain bacteria are vital in the detox process. Just about every function in the body needs enzymes. They are very delicate things, however, that are easily destroyed by the food manufacturing process, or by cooking at higher temperatures. It's the enzymes in our body that make things happen; otherwise, we would be lifeless. The correct bacteria are essential for optimum bowel function, and for encouraging good bowel flora.

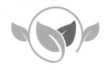

YOGHURT

Made by fermenting cow's, goat's or sheep's milk with yoghurt culture, yoghurt provides protein and calcium, and it enhances healthy gut bacteria. It is important to consume natural plain live yoghurt.

Not all yoghurts are created equal, and some flavoured yoghurt doesn't have live bacteria. The health benefits range from relieving irritable bowel syndrome to aiding digestion.

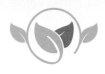

SAUERKRAUT

Sauerkraut is fermented cabbage. During the fermentation process, a method of preserving food that dates back more than 2,000 years, beneficial probiotics (or live bacteria) are produced.

These probiotics are what give sauerkraut most of its health benefits. Sauerkraut is also an acceptable form of dietary fibre, and it contains vitamins C and K, potassium, calcium and phosphorus.

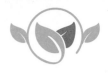

RAW FRUIT
and VEGETABLES

Fruit and vegetables are all bursting with live enzymes, and they are absolutely vital to the detoxifying process. They are also full of vitamins and minerals, plus plant compounds, making them all-powerful cleansers.

However, some are a bit better than others, and cooking them at high temperatures or for too long will destroy their delicate enzymes.

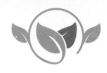

MISO

Miso means *fermented beans* in Japanese. It's a paste, traditionally made from soybeans, although you can also buy soy-free miso.

In Japan, people begin their day with a bowl of miso soup to energize the body. The protein-rich paste is an instant flavour foundation, just like stock. Rich in essential minerals and vitamins, miso provides the gut with beneficial bacteria.

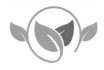

KEFIR

Kefir is like yoghurt, but it has a sharper taste. Although yoghurt is a fermented food, kefir is even better because it contains many more strains of beneficial bacteria (and some beneficial yeast), which can colonize the intestinal tract. Traditionally, kefir is made from cow's, goat's or sheep's milk.

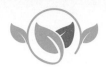

KIMCHI

Kimchi originated in Korea. It's a red, fermented cabbage dish made from a mix of salt, vinegar, garlic, chilli and other spices.

The ingredients are fermented in a tightly closed jar, and it is used as a relish, adding nutrition and probiotics to meals. Kimchi is rich in live enzymes, beneficial bacteria, vitamins and minerals.

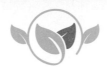

"*Let food be thy medicine, thy medicine shall be thy food.*"

HIPPOCRATES

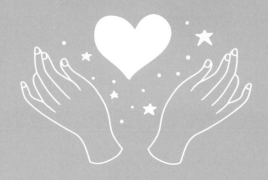

CHAPTER

5

FIBRE

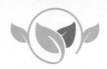

Did you know?

The term "dietary fibre" was first used in 1953 to describe the non-digestible components of plants that make up the plant cell wall. At this time, it was purely a physiological-botanical description. It was not until the 1970s that researchers started using the term in conjunction with health-related effects.

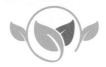

NOTES ABOUT FIBRE:

- Natural fibre from whole foods promotes good health
- Fibre provides bulk, making stools softer and more comfortable to pass
- Fibre is the perfect food for friendly bacteria
- Soluble fibre helps to lower levels of cholesterol
- Fibre speeds up the transition of waste, which ensures that autointoxication is kept to a minimum
- Fibre helps to keep our blood sugar levels stable, so less insulin is produced
- Fibre makes us feel full and therefore less likely to overeat

Many foods contain fibre, but the following are particularly good sources...

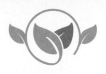

FLAXSEEDS (LINSEEDS)

These seeds are rich in lignans, which are compounds that protect against breast and ovarian cancer. They are particularly good at alleviating constipation, bloating and eliminating toxic waste from the body. They also help to reduce cholesterol levels.

Any foods that help cleanse the large intestine will drastically reduce autointoxication, which in turn will minimize fluid retention and cellulite.

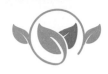

CHIA SEEDS

Chia seeds contain fibre, calcium, iron, phosphorous and antioxidants. These little seeds have a cleansing effect, and they can hold up to twelve times their weight in water. When soaked for over 30 minutes, they form a gel.

This soluble fibre acts as a prebiotic to support the growth of probiotics in the gut, balancing the bacteria.

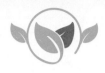

PREBIOTICS

Healthy food sources of prebiotics include tomatoes, artichokes, bananas, asparagus, onions, garlic and oats. Eating foods rich in prebiotics can keep your immune and detoxification systems healthy.

With prebiotics, good bacteria can produce nutrients called short-chain fatty acids that are beneficial for health.

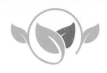

PSYLLIUM HUSKS

These ground husks contain very high levels of soluble fibre. When mixed with water, they swell and form a gel, helping stools to transit more smoothly. It bulks up the stools, encouraging the bowel to work more efficiently, so toxins are passed more quickly.

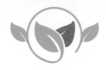

THE CASE AGAINST BRAN

You might think that bran – by which I mean wheat bran that you buy separately, or All-Bran – is good for you. However, this should be avoided as:

- It's not a whole food
- It's too concentrated
- It's too harsh for the bowel lining, often causing irritation
- It lacks nutrients
- It can contribute to dehydration
- It hinders the absorption of some vital minerals, especially iron and calcium

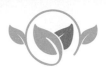

"*To keep the body in good health is a duty... otherwise we shall not be able to keep our mind strong and clear.*"

GAUTAMA BUDDHA

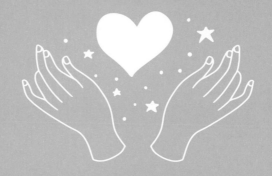

CHAPTER

6

the GUT

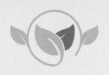

Constipation is a common complaint, and it gets worse with age. If you are constipated, you need to make solving this problem a priority, as it will have a profound effect on your overall health and detoxification.

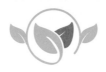

Laxatives are not a brilliant idea, as they lead to a loss of potassium and fluid, causing dehydration. Eventually, a dependency develops due to muscle weakness which ultimately *causes* constipation, which is the very thing you're trying to treat. Added to which, the laxatives themselves are toxic and the longer that waste matter stays in your bowels, the more you are poisoning yourself. Fluids are reabsorbed back into the bloodstream, giving your liver an enormous amount of extra work.

This is called autointoxication, contributing to chronic diseases, poor skin, tiredness, weight gain, headaches and accelerated ageing, to name just a few.

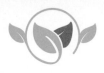

SOLVING CONSTIPATION

You will need to consume a lot more fibre from whole fruit and vegetables, from seeds like flaxseeds (linseeds) and chia seeds. Also, drink more hydrating beverages and reduce or remove those that act as diuretics (see page 13), which encourage the removal of fluids.

Also, do some gentle exercise, such as walking or yoga. Don't sit for too long and be mindful of your posture.

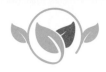

BOWEL FLORA

The intestines hold about three pounds of live bacteria that has a huge controlling influence over absorption and your general wellbeing. The environment in your intestines needs to be a little more acidic for the correct bacteria to thrive.

If too alkaline, harmful bacteria proliferate, causing a large amount of autointoxication and inflammation.

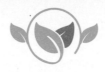

WHAT ENCOURAGES BAD OR "UNFRIENDLY" BACTERIA?

A diet with excesses of meat, wheat, sugar, milk, chocolate, tea and coffee encourages the wrong kind of bacteria, along with smoking, drinking too much alcohol, taking an excess of antibiotics or steroids, the contraceptive pill, and hormone-replacement therapy. Coupled with a lack of fresh foods like fruit and vegetables, this type of diet encourages an environment that is too alkaline, in which the unfriendly bacteria thrive and take over.

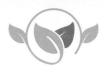

WHAT ENCOURAGES GOOD OR "FRIENDLY" BACTERIA?

A diet rich in whole, plant-based foods encourages friendly bacteria. This includes fresh fruits, vegetables, whole grains, beans, lentils and products that contain friendly bacteria like natural yoghurt, kefir, kombucha and so on. These friendly bacteria help to produce vitamins B and K, as well as generate compounds that aid and protect the immune system, contributing to good health and helping every organ in the body to detox.

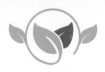

Did you know?

Our intestinal tract is actually separated from the body! Confused? Well, let me explain. The gastrointestinal mucosa forms a barrier between our external and internal world, which needs to be kept healthy, just like any other organ in the body. It is not until digested particles (molecules) pass through our intestines and into the bloodstream that they reach the inside of the body.

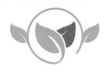

HEALTHY GUT, FEWER AUTOTOXINS

The mucosal layer needs to be healthy, otherwise optimum function is impaired, and it no longer acts as an efficient barrier/ filter between the outside and our internal environment. There is plenty of evidence to show that a leaky gut sets up food intolerances, addictions and toxins.

With the protective barrier compromised, larger molecules pass into the bloodstream that would not usually be able to do so.

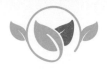

LEAKY GUT

So how does a "leaky gut" come about in the first place?

- Consuming refined, processed foods and drinks
- Drinking alcohol – e.g. more than just moderate amounts
- Medication such as antibiotics, steroids, HRT or the contraceptive pill
- Nutritional deficiencies of one type or another
- The wrong acid/alkaline environment
- Lack of enzymes, which are often due to dietary deficiencies
- Absence of the correct fibre intake
- Sometimes chemotherapy
- Certain auto-immune diseases

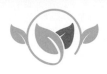

"All disease begins in the gut."

HIPPOCRATES

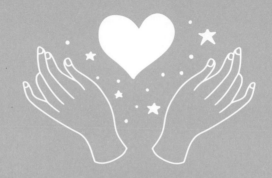

CHAPTER
7

SUPPLEMENTS

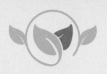

If you want to detox, you need to focus on eating and drinking the right kind of food. This way, you will have more energy, improved metabolism, less fluid retention, organs that function efficiently, less constipation and so on. Supplements should be thought of as the icing on the cake – nice to have, but not essential. Just as a car works well when all the parts are in sync, the same goes for the human body.

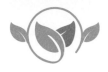

ALPHA LIPOIC ACID (ALA)

ALA is often referred to as the *universal antioxidant*. That's because, unusually, it is both fat- and water-soluble, allowing it to enter all parts of the body to neutralize free radicals.

This is important because toxins are stored in fat cells. It can also help regenerate vitamin E, vitamin C and help the liver function to detox more efficiently.

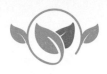

LECITHIN

A natural substance found in egg yolks,
soybeans and sunflower seeds, lecithin
is unique because it is fat- and water-
soluble. One of the liver's key roles is
to break down fat-soluble toxins into
water-soluble ones, making them more
comfortable and safer to excrete.
Phosphatidylcholine in lecithin works
in the liver to strengthen liver cells by
making their outer membrane strong and
resistant to the infiltration of toxins.

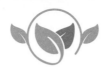

VITAMIN C

Vitamin C helps the body manufacture glutathione, which allows the liver to detox. Research has shown that as little as 500mg of vitamin C raised levels of glutathione by 50 per cent in just two weeks. Vitamins C is also a powerful antioxidant. Fruit and vegetables are packed with vitamin C, but too much cooking will destroy it. If you feel you are not getting a sufficient amount through your diet, add 1000–2000mg capsules or tablets daily.

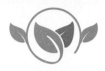

Did you know?

Most animals can make their own vitamin C, but we are among the few that can't, so we need to take it in from foods or sometimes supplements as well. The other animals that can't make their own vitamin C are bats, guinea pigs, apes and monkeys.

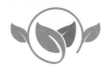

PROBIOTICS

It is challenging to maintain a good gut flora due to the toxins, medications and chemicals that we are exposed to daily; antibiotics, food preservatives, pesticides and chlorinated water all help to destroy good bacteria.

Even people suffering from chronic stress will have an imbalance of good bacteria. Taking probiotics and a change in diet can help improve matters.

MSM

Methylsulphonylmethane (MSM), a chemical found in green plants, animals and humans and available as a supplement, contains biologically active sulphur, which is necessary for many critical bodily functions, including detoxification.

MSM helps facilitate the detoxification process by making cells more permeable, which helps to release built-up heavy metals, waste and toxins. This also makes it easier for nutrients and water to enter the cells and continue the cleansing process.

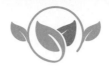

CHLORELLA

This blue-green algae is a natural *chelator* – meaning it can bind to heavy metal toxins in the body and keep them from being reabsorbed while being expelled.

This is especially important for those with mercury fillings, those who have been vaccinated, or who eat fish regularly. The high levels of chlorophyll in chlorella protect the body against ultraviolet radiation treatments while removing radioactive particles from the body.

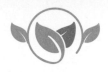

FULVIC ACID

Fulvic acid is known to boost digestion, improve nutrient absorption and gut health. It's found naturally in the soil and works by stimulating the good bacteria in the intestines.

Fulvic acid helps restore the body's ideal acid/alkali level, which further hinders the growth and proliferation of harmful bacteria, yeasts, fungi and other microorganisms. This cuts down the toxins the body must deal with.

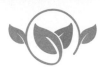

REISHI MUSHROOM

Rich in antioxidants, this mushroom has been used medicinally for thousands of years – it is so vital that it is called the *king of mushrooms*.

Chinese medicine focuses on disease prevention instead of treatment, so the emphasis is on the liver, as it is the organ responsible for cleaning, processing and circulating healthy blood and nutrients.

SCHISANDRA

A medicinal berry that has been used for thousands of years in Traditional Chinese Medicine, schisandra is probably best known for its impact on the liver and adrenal function. It boosts the production of various detoxifying enzymes, while also balancing hormones naturally, supporting the adrenal glands, which help the body deal with stress.

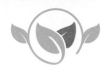

GLUTATHIONE

Glutathione engages in making DNA, the building blocks of proteins and cells, supporting immune function and breaking down some free radicals. It helps certain enzymes function, transports mercury out of the brain, allowing the liver and gallbladder to deal with fats and toxins.

Reducing toxin exposure and increasing your intake of healthful foods are also excellent ways to naturally increase glutathione levels.

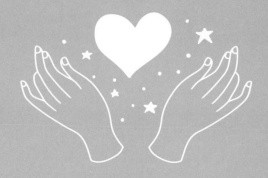

CHAPTER

8

SPROUTS
and
SPROUTING

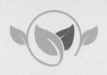

While sprouting,
seeds, grains, beans or
lentils burst into life and
their nutritional content
increases hugely –
especially enzymes – in a
matter of days. Sprouting
them also makes them
much easier to digest and
assimilate.

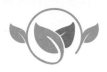

So, if you have trouble digesting beans, sprouting will make all the difference.

The method is so simple; anyone can get impressive results with minimal effort. Sprouts can be added to salads, sandwiches, wraps, smoothies, chopped in dips, very lightly steamed or added to a stir-fry at the end of cooking. Avoid cooking sprouts too much, however, or you risk destroying their delicate enzymes.

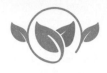

HOW TO SPROUT

Method 1

Soak two heaped tablespoons of the beans, lentils or grains listed on page 116 (one heaped tablespoon for seeds) in water overnight and then discard the water. In about three to five days, the sprouts should be ready. Wash well, drain and store in the fridge, consume as soon as possible (within three days is best).

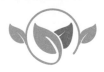

Method 2

Place the soaked grains or seeds in a large glass jar. Don't put too many in because they need room to expand and grow. Place a piece of netting over the opening of the jar and secure it with an elastic band. Pour water in through the mesh and, importantly, pour the water out again. Do this twice a day. DO NOT leave sprouts sitting in water, as they will rot.

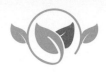

Method 3

Buy or make sprouting sacks, which have a drawstring top and are made from 100 per cent loose-weave linen or hemp, as these fabrics don't rot. Place the soaked grains or seeds into the sack, then drop the sack into some clean water. Immediately hang the sack up over the sink, allowing the sprouts to drain. Rinse them in water twice a day.

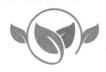

Method 4

This method is similar to the previous one, but instead of a sack, place the soaked grains or seeds into a basket, put the basket into the water and hang it up over the sink, allowing the basket to drain. Do this twice a day. Cover the basket with a tea towel to keep flies and dust off your sprouts.

what can be
SPROUTED?

All sorts of seeds, grains and legumes – including lentils, chickpeas, sesame, sunflower seeds, alfalfa, mung beans (bean shoots), broccoli seed, radish seeds, fenugreek seeds or whole grains like spelt or kamut. For very little time and effort, you will have fresh, detoxifying, enzyme- and nutrient-rich food available all year round at a fraction of the price of buying sprouts.

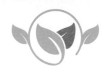

ALFALFA SPROUTS

This sprout is high in a plant fibre called plant plantix, giving it the ability to bind to some toxins such as chemical food additives. Alfalfa is also a rich source of vitamins, minerals and amino acids.

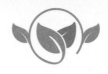

SPROUTED FENUGREEK SEEDS

These seeds were held in high regard by the Egyptians, Greeks and Romans. They smell a little like celery but have a mild, bitter/sour taste. Excellent for improving fluid retention and cellulite, studies have shown that fenugreek seeds can also help stabilize blood sugar levels. In addition, they help clear lymph and ease muscle spasms, period pains, stomach cramps and heavy legs.

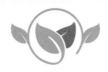

SPROUTED MUNG BEANS

Rich in essential amino acids, sprouting mung beans reduce levels of phytic acid, which is an anti-nutrient. Mung beans also contain something called resistant starch, which works similarly to soluble fibre, helping to nourish your good bacteria.

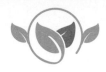

BROCCOLI SPROUTS

Broccoli sprouts are a rich source of glucoraphanin, which is a precursor to the potent phytochemical sulforaphane.

Sulforaphane initiates phase-two liver detoxification, the stage when the liver converts toxic metabolites into less-toxic compounds, which are then ready for excretion. It also dramatically increases glutathione, the body's primary antioxidant and detoxifier.

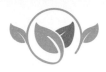

RADISHES

Like other vegetables of the brassica family (cabbage, broccoli, Brussels sprouts and the like), radishes contain two natural compounds – sulforaphane and indole-3 – prompting the body to make higher levels of detoxifying enzymes.

Radishes help the liver do a better job of breaking down harmful substances into less harmful ones, and they contain a significant amount of vitamin C to boost defence against disease.

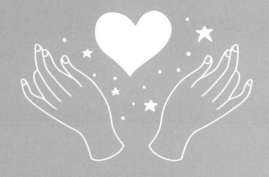

CHAPTER
9

LIMITING TOXIC EXPOSURES

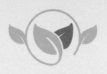

We are surrounded by
a toxic chemical cocktail. Still,
it is not all doom and gloom,
because we can reduce our
exposure dramatically. There
are toxins that we voluntarily
consume or inhale such as
alcohol, nicotine, caffeine,
room fresheners, sprays or
chemical food additives.
Always remember to check
the labels and ingredients
before you buy.

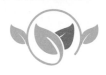

"If organic farming is the natural way, shouldn't organic produce just be called produce and make the pesticide-laden stuff take the burden of an adjective?"

YMBER DELECTO

TOXINS and
your BODY

Although exposure to toxins is almost unavoidable and the sources can be anything from environmental exposure to pesticides on food, we can reduce negative effects by making good dietary and lifestyle choices.

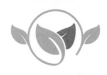

ORGANIC FOOD

Eating organic food has many benefits. Besides being more sustainable and better for the environment, eating organic food will help minimize your intake of toxic pesticides and herbicides.

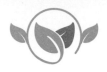

ALCOHOL

There is no completely safe level of drinking alcohol. If you regularly drink more than three units of alcohol a day, you are at risk of causing major organ damage, or at the very least hindering organ function.

Binge drinking can have a detrimental effect on the organs over time.

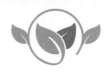

CAFFEINE

A lot of people find it hard to give up caffeine because it is addictive. In some people, as little as 350 grams has been shown to lower concentration levels.

Caffeine is a stimulant, but you can suffer from fatigue unless you keep taking in more, so a dependency develops and you end up needing more and more of it to feel normal.

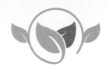

SALT

Consuming too much salt can cause your body to retain excess fluid, and this is worse if you don't drink enough water. This encourages the body to release an antidiuretic hormone that prevents you from urinating and from detoxing.

By decreasing salt intake and increasing your water intake, the body reduces the secretion of this hormone and it increases urination, which means you eliminate more water and waste products.

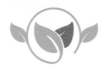

SUGAR

During research to discover which foods caused the most significant free radical damage, sugar was found to be the worst! Within two hours of eating 300 grams of sugar, which is equivalent to a can of fizzy drink, free radicals increased by 140 per cent. Also, the levels of the harmful bacteria went up, raising the possibility of more toxins being reabsorbed.

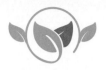

Did you know?

The average American consumes seven times as much sugar as the average British person, but even the Brits consume too much. In France, 53 per cent of the population eat cake, while nearly 40 per cent of Europeans eat chocolate when stressed. Sugar is everywhere and in everything, and it takes an effort to avoid it, but it can be done.

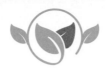

STRESS

When you become stressed, the body produces a variety of chemicals that put it into a state of alert, and these extra chemicals need to be broken down by the organs. Plus, being stressed means you are more likely to eat the foods that cause toxicity.

TOXINS in the HOME

Substituting natural ingredients for chemical cleaning products or buying eco-friendly home alternatives can go a long way towards reducing your exposure to toxins in the home.

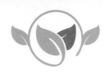

PERSONAL CARE PRODUCTS

A good deal of whatever you put on your skin is absorbed into the bloodstream, so it's a good idea to change your personal care products to those with natural ingredients.

AIR FRESHENERS

Air fresheners, room sprays and room plug-ins pollute the home and ensure that you and your loved ones inhale them.

Change to pure, 100 per cent natural, therapeutic essential oils. Heat them in an oil diffuser or room-therapy air fresheners. Mix a few drops of essential oil into a bowl of bicarbonate of soda and leave out as an air-freshener.

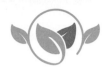

CARPET FRESHENER

Bicarbonate of soda or baking powder is particularly useful for absorbing odours. Sprinkle some over the carpet and then brush it in, leaving it for a few minutes before vacuuming it up.

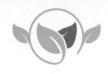

WINDOW CLEANER

Fill a spray bottle with equal amounts of vinegar and water. You can add a little washing-up liquid if you wish, then spray the windows and wipe clean with a cloth.

Alternatively, use some cleaning alcohol. Simply spray the windows and wipe clean.

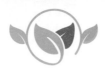

FLOOR CLEANER

Add half a cup of vinegar to one gallon of hot water and mop the floor.
You can buy clear, distilled white vinegar very inexpensively. Alternatively, add a little eco-friendly soap to a bucket of hot water.

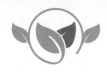

TOILET CLEANER

Use vinegar instead of a chemical cleaner by putting it into a spray bottle. Spray the toilet and leave for at least ten minutes while it kills germs and deodorizes simultaneously.

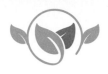

*"We are living in
a world today where
lemonade is made from
artificial flavours, and
furniture polish is made
from real lemons!"*

ALFRED E. NEWMAN

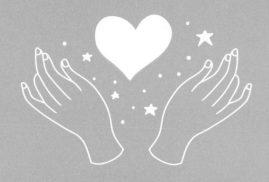

CHAPTER
10

SIDE EFFECTS of DETOXING

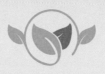

For most people, side effects after starting a detox are inevitable. The number of side effects people suffer will vary from person to person, and some will suffer more intensely than others. To reduce some of these feelings, incorporate some of the suggestions listed in Chapter 11 and try some professional treatments. The good thing about side effects is that they are temporary; some may only last a day or so, while others may stick around for a week, so don't give up.

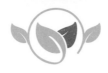

HEADACHES

Whether you decide to go "cold turkey" or gradually cut back, most people have experienced the headache or even migraine that comes with giving up caffeine in tea, coffee or soft drinks.

Luckily, it's temporary, lasting about two days for some and a few days more for others. Usually the blood vessels in the brain constrict, but when we remove caffeine, they dilate.

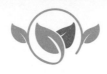

DIGESTIVE PROBLEMS

These are common on a detox diet. When we consume fresh whole foods, fruit and vegetables, we are taking in more than the usual amount of fibre. With this extra fibre, some people experience cramps, while others might get diarrhoea. On the other hand, if you are giving up caffeine or cigarettes, you might experience constipation, because coffee and nicotine stimulate the bowels.

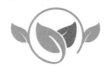

SKIN PROBLEMS

The skin is our largest detoxing organ, and as a result you might get a rash, itching or spots upon embarking on a detox diet. It is possible that you might experience some sweating and a bad smell, even after bathing or showering. It shouldn't last too long, however; as you continue to improve your health, the other organs will work more efficiently, thus taking the pressure off the skin.

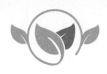

INCREASED URINATION

Frequent trips to the bathroom are common with detoxes. A lot of people are intolerant of the chemicals in processed foods such as preservatives, colourings, enhancers and so on. The body will try to conserve fluids to dilute the foods that are causing irritation, so when you remove these foods, you may urinate more. However, this can also be due to taking in more of the hydrating fluids.

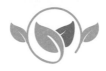

EXISTING CONDITIONS

A few people's pre-existing conditions temporarily worsen before they improve on a detox. Eczema or rashes, aches and pains may increase for a short time, or you may experience fatigue, depression and more.

If the reaction is severe, slow down the process by continuing to eat some of the wrong kinds of things as well as the right ones for a while.

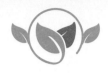

TIP for LOW ENERGY

Research has shown that ginkgo biloba, which is found in supplements, helps boost people's mental energy and concentration. Read the instructions on the bottle and only take the recommended dose.

This is not a detox herb, but it might help combat temporary energy lows.

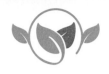

"*Our bodies
are our gardens –
our wills are our
gardeners.*"

WILLIAM SHAKESPEARE

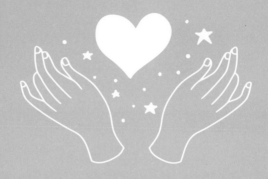

CHAPTER
11

DO-IT-
YOURSELF
TREATMENTS

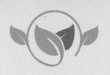

There are many
treatments you can do
at home to enhance the
detox process and reduce
side effects. Incorporate
some of those listed in
the following pages, and
you will soon feel better.
Most require products
that are easy to find and
simple to manage.

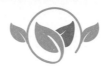

DRY SKIN BRUSHING

The skin is the largest elimination organ, sometimes referred to as the third kidney. Dry skin brushing with a natural bristle brush is a powerful way to enhance the detoxification process. It improves the appearance of your skin, stimulating the blood circulation and, most importantly, the lymphatic system.

Brush the body lightly in long, smooth strokes, always working towards the heart.

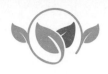

EPSOM SALTS

Put some Epsom salts (magnesium sulphate) in your bathtub. If you don't have a bathtub, a foot bath or a large bowl filled with warm water and a little Epsom salt works well too.

For strong detoxing, dissolve half a pound or about 250 kilograms in a hot bath and soak for a minimum of 20–30 minutes, long enough for the body to absorb the magnesium it needs.

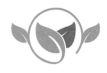

ESSENTIAL OIL BATHS

Essential oil baths help the body relax and detox. Run a hot bath, put on some relaxing music, light some candles, leave your phone in another room and close the door. Add eight drops of essential oil and agitate the water surface before getting in the bath.

Relax, breathe in the aroma and soak for 20–30 minutes, allowing the skin to absorb the therapeutic properties.

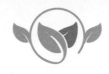

CASTOR OIL PACK
(External Use Only)

Castor oil contains protein-like compounds that stimulate immune responses, helping to break down toxic build-up. Fold a piece of natural cotton and soak it with castor oil. Place it on the area to be treated, which may be the liver or a painful joint. Cover the cotton with a piece of cling film and place a hot-water bottle or heat pad over it. Leave it in place for 30–60 minutes.

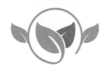

SALT SCRUB

Mix one cup of finely ground sea salt with some glycerine to make a paste. Then add five drops of pure lemon essential oil. Stand in the shower and rub the salt mixture into your body – avoiding any broken skin – before showering it off.

You will exfoliate and improve your circulation and lymph flow.

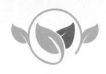

SWEATING

Anything that causes sweating will help the body detox quicker and more efficiently. One of the obvious ways to do this is exercise, of course. I know so many people who hate the E word, however, so here is an alternative.

Take a hot bath while drinking hot ginger tea, then go to bed with a couple of hot-water bottles and cover yourself with lots of layers.

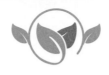

TAKE A WALK

Walking helps the detox process by getting the circulation and lymph moving. It also allows you to detox via the lungs as you breathe more deeply and get fresh air. A 20-minute walk every day is meant to be all you need.

The best places to walk are in the countryside or in a park where there are plenty of trees.

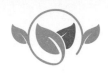

ENEMAS

If you suffer from chronic constipation, then you might consider kick-starting your detox program with an enema. Still, as you change your diet, your bowels should begin to function more efficiently on their own.

However, if you decide on an enema, there is plenty of information online about how to use an enema kit, which you can buy at a pharmacy or online.

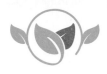

'The best six doctors anywhere

And no one can deny it

Are sunshine, water, rest and air,

Exercise and diet.'

Nursery rhyme quoted by WAYNE FIELDS,
What the River Knows (1990)

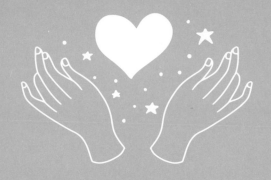

CHAPTER
12

TREATMENTS
and
PRACTICES

Several natural treatments will help enhance the body's detoxing process. These will go a long way to relieving side effects by giving your body a helping hand.

One of the nicest and, indeed, the most relaxing is to have a massage, as this helps improve circulation. Research has shown that when the body is massaged, the skin's temperature rises. This widens the gaps between cells, allowing for better lymph flow. It also reduces stress.

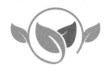

LYMPHATIC MASSAGE

Lymphatic drainage technique is the most beneficial of all the massages for detoxing the lymph. Long, soft, gentle sweeping movements are used.

A specialist must perform this technique to be effective, as it is achieved in a specific sequence.

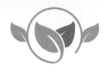

STEAM AND SAUNA

Anything that helps the body sweat is useful for getting rid of stored toxins. If you change your diet to one that involves fresh, natural foods and drinks, the cells eliminate more waste and toxins into the bloodstream for the organs to handle.

Anything you can do to speed up the process and take the pressure off the organs, the better you will feel.

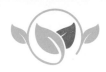

ACUPUNCTURE

An acupuncturist uses super-thin needles, positioned in the right combination of specific points on the body, to stimulate positive energy flow and create balance between organs and systems.

Natural detoxification by use of acupuncture is effective because it treats the entire body, along with the mental, spiritual and emotional areas.

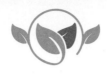

AROMATHERAPY

The application of specific essential oils dilated in a carrier oil greatly enhances the detox process. The oils enter the bloodstream through the skin and through the nose. What a lovely way to detox!

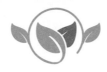

YOGA and TAI CHI

These exercise regimes help you to breathe properly, leading to better-functioning lungs and more efficient detoxing. Stretching the muscles helps release tension, stored lactic acid and other toxins.

Reducing stress makes a significant difference as the body produces fewer stress hormones, which are ultimately toxic. Yoga also stimulates the lymphatic system, contracting and relaxing the muscles to boost the flow around the body.

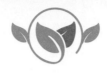

FULL-BODY WRAP

Body wraps, also known as body masks, use detoxifying algae, mud or clay to help draw out toxins from the skin.

As the skin is your largest organ, this can have a significant effect on your health and overall wellbeing. The body is first exfoliated, which helps stimulate the circulation and remove dead cells. This treatment also encourages sweating.

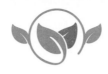

IV INFUSIONS

These have become very popular, with intravenous studios popping up everywhere, even in beauty salons. People are having nutritive IVs if their immune system is run down, if they are suffering from stress or low energy levels or if they wish to detox.

Some people even take them for a hangover, as it is a quick way to hydrate and get vitamin C and other nutrients into the system.

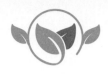

*"What fools indeed
we mortals are
To lavish care upon a car,
With ne'er a bit of
time to see
About our own
machinery!"*

JOHN KENDRICK BANGS

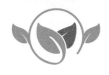

"The part can never be well unless the whole is well."

PLATO

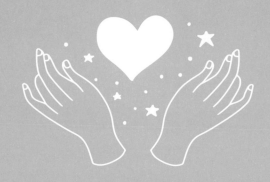

CHAPTER
13

DE-CLUTTER

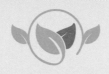

It's essential to have a good spring clean and de-clutter as part of your detox plan. This will clear your mind and many other areas of your life that could do with cleansing and detoxing. Organize your kitchen cupboards, sort out your wardrobes, and this will ease some of the stress in your daily life. Clear your office of unwanted papers, magazines and junk, and detox every part of your life for a healthier, happier you.

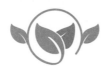

KITCHEN
CUPBOARDS

Before you start on your detox adventure, start with giving your kitchen cupboards a good clear-out. Most people find out-of-date products hiding in there, but, more importantly, there will be food that won't be suitable to eat after you have carried out your detox programme.

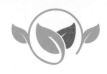

WARDROBE
and DRAWERS

Many of us have a wardrobe full of clothes that we haven't worn for a long time and that we probably never will. Some clothes need to be repaired, but it is hard to see what we actually have when the wardrobe is crammed full.

Take everything out and go through each item. Sort your stuff into four piles: one pile to keep, one to repair, one for charity and another to throw away.

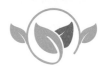

ROOM by ROOM

Go through each room and decide what you don't need any longer and give it away or sell it. Getting rid of unneeded belongings will make it easier to clean each room. Invest in a good vacuum cleaner with a HEPA filter. Vacuum the curtains, carpets, furniture and mattresses really well.

All vacuums come with all sorts of attachments these days – why not challenge yourself to use them all!

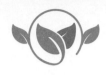

OPEN WINDOWS

Open the windows as often as you can, depending on the weather, and let fresh air blow through the rooms.

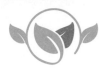

the MIND

Try to reduce stress and de-clutter your mind while detoxing. To do this, set a goal to reduce the time you spend on social media. Or set time aside when you don't answer the phone or react to messages.

Detox by getting into the habit of off-loading into a notebook physically or electronically. This way, you don't need to juggle all those things that you have to remember, which take up your precious time and energy.

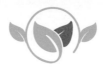

CHECKLIST

Consider what is making you stressed and think about things that are harmful to your mind and body. Is it money, your job, your relationship or your friends?

Whatever it is, find out what you can do about it. Can you change your career or talk to your boss, or simply change your attitude towards it?

Work out a budget and see how you can increase income or save money. Reduce time spent with toxic family members and dump jealous and destructive friends right now.

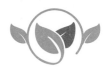

HOBBIES

Learn to embroider or knit, do jigsaw puzzles, read or cook. There are so many hobbies to choose from; the list is endless. Find a space that is dedicated to your hobby or set time aside for your amusement. Make sure you have some time to be quiet.

A friend of mine grows much of the salad, fruit and vegetables that she and her family eat, so she says her garden is her gym and her de-stress area.

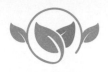

DE-STRESS
JOURNAL

Journals have been proven to be extremely useful as a de-stressing and healing tool. Journals come in all sorts of styles and mediums. You can use them to say what you think, feel and are grateful for, what's happened in your day, what needs to go and so much more.

Remember, whatever you choose, don't look for perfection, as this might stress you out and defeat the object of the exercise.

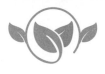

MAKE A LIST

Write things down, make bullet points or create a list. This could be a list of things you love or are grateful for, or a to-do list, or anything in between. A food journal is especially useful when starting a detox and a new, healthier life.

Keep track of the supplements you take, the side effects and your weight. You could even note down new recipes that you like. Make your comments enjoyable by using colour-coded markers or adding symbols.

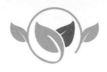

BE ARTSY

My favourite way to de-stress is working in an art journal. I am not an artist – far from it – but drawing simple things from everyday life can help in so many ways.

You will need an art journal, pencil, eraser, sharpener, coloured pencils or watercolour and a couple of pens with permanent black ink. Check online; you will see hundreds of examples to give you an idea of how to start.

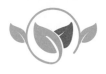

"Your body is precious. It is our vehicle for awakening. Treat it with care."

GAUTAMA BUDDHA

CONCLUSION

You might like to think about what you will do after your detox. Whether you choose to follow a specific diet, such as raw or keto, vegan or macrobiotic, the most important aspect to consider is avoiding anything that is processed or refined. Additionally, stay away from food that contains chemicals, too much sugar or gluten and choose products that are natural, whole and organic if possible. If you wish to include meat, eat less of it and try to buy organic or free-range products. Hydrate and have fermented food regularly. You don't need to follow a specific diet, but if you need help, consult a naturopath or nutritional therapist.

Whatever you do, don't put all that effort to waste. Detoxing is the start of a healthier lifestyle that will result in fewer unpleasant reactions to foods and the products that surround us. After a detox, we have more energy, sleep better, have more patience and look nicer, so it really is a beneficial thing to do, especially if it is followed up by a healthier lifestyle.

Good luck
Sonia

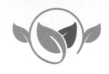

"Every human being is the author of his own health or disease."

GAUTAMA BUDDHA